SUZANNE BYRD

ADHD and Organisation: A Woman's Perspective

Contents

1

Understanding ADHD in Women

Introduction

ADHD is often associated with hyperactive, restless boys, but for many women, ADHD shows up in unique ways, often under the radar. Women with ADHD are frequently undiagnosed until adulthood, as symptoms can present differently. This chapter aims to shed light on ADHD as it affects women and introduces the reader to strategies tailored to their needs.

Why ADHD Can Look Different in Women

Research indicates that women often experience ADHD as a more internalized condition. Rather than the stereotypical "can't sit still" behavior, women may face intense emotional shifts, a feeling of "brain fog," and a persistent sense of being overwhelmed by daily tasks. Hormonal fluctuations can exacerbate ADHD symptoms, impacting focus and emotional regulation.

The Journey to Diagnosis

For many women, the path to an ADHD diagnosis is long and winding. They may not receive an official diagnosis until well into adulthood, often after recognizing patterns of struggle that friends or family members don't seem to share. These challenges can manifest in various ways: a consistent feeling of underachievement, disorganization, procrastination, and a sense of being "different." Many women who seek diagnosis do so after learning about ADHD through friends or reading, recognizing their struggles in the experiences of others.

Take, for example, Sarah's Story: Sarah, a 34-year-old project manager and mother of two, always felt she was barely managing to stay on top of her responsibilities. She struggled to organize her tasks at work, frequently losing track of deadlines. At home, she found it impossible to keep up with household chores and was constantly frustrated by the feeling that her brain was scattered. It wasn't until a friend mentioned her own recent ADHD diagnosis that Sarah began researching the condition and realized that many of her daily challenges could be attributed to ADHD.

Sarah's experience of finally understanding herself through an ADHD lens was transformative. It allowed her to forgive herself for years of struggle, embrace the reality of her brain's unique wiring, and, more importantly, take actionable steps toward managing her symptoms.

Common Organizational Challenges for Women with ADHD

ADHD can make organization particularly challenging for women, especially when they juggle multiple roles, such as career responsibilities, family duties, and personal goals. For many, the demands of life create a perpetual state of "too much to do, too little time" — a feeling heightened by ADHD.

Here are a few common organizational challenges faced by women with ADHD:

Executive Function Difficulties: Planning, prioritizing, and decision-making are tasks managed by executive functions in the brain, which are often weaker in those with ADHD.

Time Blindness: Many women with ADHD struggle with an altered sense of time. They may underestimate how long tasks will take, leading to chronic lateness or last-minute rushes.

Emotional Sensitivity: The emotional component of ADHD can create challenges in personal and professional relationships, leading to feelings of guilt, shame, and low self-worth.

Perfectionism and Procrastination: Women with ADHD often experience a paradox of perfectionism and procrastination, where they delay tasks because they feel they won't meet their own high standards.

Understanding these challenges is the first step toward managing them, and that's exactly what this book aims to achieve. Each of the following chapters will dive into practical strategies to tackle specific issues, allowing readers to develop an ADHD-

3

friendly approach to organization.

Practical Tips to Start Your Journey

To begin with, here are a few starter strategies that have worked for women managing ADHD:

1. Self-Acceptance and Compassion: Begin by accepting that your brain processes information differently. Women like Sarah often find relief in understanding that ADHD isn't a lack of effort but a neurological difference. Being kind to yourself can reduce the pressure to "be perfect" and help you move forward with realistic expectations.

2. Breaking Down Tasks: For women with ADHD, tasks that feel overwhelming can lead to paralysis. One way to combat this is to break tasks down into smaller, manageable steps. For example, instead of writing "clean the kitchen" on your to-do list, break it down into "wash dishes," "wipe counters," and "empty trash."

3. Setting Visual Cues: Many women with ADHD find visual cues helpful, such as using sticky notes or setting reminders on their phones. This makes it easier to stay on top of tasks and prevents important things from falling through the cracks.

4. Embracing the Power of a Timer: Timers can be life-changing for managing ADHD. Setting a timer for 10-15 minutes to tackle a

specific task helps create a sense of urgency and provides a clear start and end point. This is particularly useful for overcoming "task inertia" — the resistance to starting something you know you need to do.

5. Celebrating Small Wins: Recognizing and celebrating even small accomplishments can create positive reinforcement and keep you motivated. ADHD often skews our sense of self-worth, so taking time to appreciate your progress can boost your morale and build momentum.

Reflection

Understanding ADHD is crucial for developing effective strategies that work with your brain rather than against it. Through Sarah's story, we see the importance of compassion and self-understanding in the ADHD journey. Women facing ADHD often carry years of shame and frustration; however, recognizing and accepting their ADHD can be an incredibly empowering first step.

In the following chapters, we'll explore specific strategies that work in a variety of areas, from creating routines to managing time and finances. Each chapter will include actionable ideas tailored for women, along with real-life case studies to demonstrate how these strategies have helped others. Together, we'll build a toolkit to help you thrive, navigate daily life with confidence, and embrace the strengths ADHD can bring.

2

Building A Supportive Environment

One of the most critical components of managing ADHD is creating a supportive environment. This includes both physical spaces that are conducive to focus and mental spaces filled with people who understand and uplift you. Building a supportive environment can make the difference between feeling constantly overwhelmed and feeling empowered to tackle your goals. This chapter will dive into practical methods for cultivating spaces and relationships that help, rather than hinder, productivity and mental health.

Why a Supportive Environment Matters

For women with ADHD, a supportive environment isn't just a nice-to-have; it's a necessity. ADHD often brings challenges in focus, organization, and memory, which can feel exacerbated in an environment that's chaotic or unsupportive. Physical and social environments that are attuned to ADHD needs can alleviate stress, reduce feelings of isolation, and provide helpful accountability.

Consider Maria's Story: Maria, a busy entrepreneur, found herself struggling to stay organized and meet deadlines. She would get lost in ideas, working on half a dozen projects at once and losing track of her priorities. Maria knew she needed a change but didn't know where to start. After attending an ADHD support group, she learned about the importance of supportive environments. She began to cultivate a small group of people who helped keep her on track and started working in spaces designed to minimize distractions.

Maria's journey shows that environment can either amplify ADHD challenges or help mitigate them. Through thoughtful adjustments, she transformed her work habits, ultimately finding balance and increasing her productivity.

Building a Physical Space That Supports Focus

A chaotic or cluttered space can be a significant source of distraction for those with ADHD. Crafting an environment that's clean, simple, and supportive of focus can create a strong foundation for productivity.

1. Create Clear Zones: Establish specific areas for different activities. For example, designate one area for work, another for relaxation, and another for daily tasks like bill-paying or planning. Clear zones help create a mental association, so you're more likely to focus on the task at hand.

2. Limit Visual Clutter: Too many visual stimuli can be overwhelming for the ADHD brain. Try keeping only essential items

on your desk or workspace and removing unnecessary objects. Use storage containers and drawers to keep things out of sight but easily accessible.

3. Add Visual Reminders: Visual cues can also be helpful if they are intentional and limited. For instance, placing a sticky note with your top three tasks for the day in your workspace can keep you focused on priorities.

4. Utilize Whiteboards or Bulletin Boards: For some women with ADHD, having a physical space to map out tasks and ideas is helpful. Use a whiteboard or bulletin board to organize ongoing projects and to-do lists visually, helping you stay on track.

5. Incorporate Comfort Elements: Because sensory overload is common, think about making your space comfortable with soft lighting, a good chair, and minimal noise. Noise-canceling headphones can also help if you're sensitive to sound.

Creating a Social Environment That Empowers You

Your social circle can greatly impact your ability to manage ADHD. Surrounding yourself with people who understand your challenges, support your goals, and help keep you accountable can provide a steady foundation for growth.

1. Seek Out Accountability Partners: Find a friend or family member willing to help you stay on track. They don't have to

manage or micromanage you; sometimes, just knowing you'll report back to someone can improve follow-through.

2. Join ADHD Support Groups: Connecting with others who share similar experiences can reduce feelings of isolation and provide fresh perspectives. ADHD support groups, whether online or in person, offer a safe space to exchange ideas, share struggles, and find encouragement.

3. Educate Close Friends and Family: Many people misunderstand ADHD, so it's important to have honest conversations with those closest to you about what ADHD is and how it affects your life. Setting expectations can help prevent frustration and foster a more supportive dynamic.

4. Set Boundaries: Boundaries are essential, especially for women who are often expected to juggle multiple roles. Politely but firmly setting limits can protect your time and energy for your most important tasks.

Case Study: Anna's Accountability Network

Anna, a 29-year-old marketing manager, found herself struggling to meet deadlines despite her best efforts. She often felt judged by her family and friends, who didn't understand the unique challenges of her ADHD. After a difficult conversation with her sister, she decided to reach out to a few close friends and ask them for support, sharing her experience and needs honestly. Her friends agreed to help her stay accountable, not through constant check-ins but with regular catch-ups where she could review her progress and receive encouragement.

Over time, Anna's productivity increased, and so did her confidence. Her friends gained a better understanding of her experience with ADHD and became part of her support system. This network helped Anna reframe her relationship with ADHD, making her feel less alone and more capable.

Building a Supportive Routine for Mental Health

Mental health is a key component of a supportive environment, especially for women with ADHD. Establishing routines that prioritize self-care can help reduce stress and build resilience.

1. Incorporate Downtime: Schedule time to unwind and disconnect. Even if it's just a 15-minute break, taking time to recharge is essential to avoid burnout.

2. Practice Mindfulness Techniques: Simple practices like deep breathing, meditation, or short yoga sessions can help center your mind and manage impulsivity.

3. Set Realistic Expectations: Many women with ADHD struggle with perfectionism, leading to feelings of inadequacy. Setting small, realistic goals and allowing room for mistakes can make routines sustainable.

4. Check in with Yourself Regularly: Try to reflect daily or weekly

on your environment, identifying what's working and what isn't. Make adjustments as necessary, prioritizing changes that will create the most positive impact.

Reflection

Creating a supportive environment—both physical and social—is a powerful strategy for managing ADHD effectively. Just as we saw with Maria and Anna, building an environment that caters to your unique needs can alleviate stress, improve productivity, and help you thrive.

Remember that this process takes time. You may need to experiment with different setups and connections to find what works best. The most important part is to make intentional choices about your environment and the people in your life, ensuring they contribute positively to your well-being and goals.

In the next chapter, we'll explore "The Power of Routine," examining how consistent habits can anchor your day and provide structure amidst the challenges of ADHD. Through practical tips and real-life stories, you'll discover how to create routines that work with your ADHD, not against it.

3

The Power of Routine

For women with ADHD, routines can serve as an invaluable anchor. Many women with ADHD feel overwhelmed by the chaos of daily life, but routines offer a way to regain control and provide a sense of predictability. They create a rhythm that reduces anxiety, helps manage time effectively, and fosters a sense of accomplishment. This chapter will provide strategies for establishing routines that support focus, minimize distractions, and, most importantly, work with the ADHD brain.

Why Routines Matter for ADHD

Routine is powerful because it reduces the need for constant decision-making. For those with ADHD, the mental fatigue that comes from making countless small decisions throughout the day can be overwhelming. A routine simplifies this process by providing a predictable structure. With repetition, these routines can become almost automatic, allowing you to focus on what matters without being sidetracked by minor decisions or distractions.

Let's look at Emma's Story: Emma, a 42-year-old teacher, used to feel like her day was constantly slipping away. She'd start the morning with grand plans but soon found herself overwhelmed by competing demands. After a series of trial-and-error attempts, she developed a morning and evening routine that provided the structure she needed. Her mornings began with 10 minutes of planning, where she identified her top three priorities. At night, she had a routine of winding down, reviewing the day, and preparing for the next.

Emma found that even a simple routine brought her more clarity and control, making her feel grounded despite her busy life.

Steps to Build a Routine That Works for You

Building a routine doesn't mean creating a rigid schedule that feels impossible to follow. Flexibility is key, especially for women with ADHD. Here are steps to help create a routine that aligns with your lifestyle and ADHD needs:

1. Start Small: Attempting a drastic overhaul is likely to backfire. Instead, start with a single habit that you'd like to incorporate into your day. For example, if mornings are difficult, begin by establishing just one small action that brings calm, such as spending five minutes stretching or setting priorities for the day.

2. Use "Anchor" Activities: Many people with ADHD find it helpful to attach a new routine to an existing habit. For instance, if you always make coffee in the morning, use that time to check your calendar or write down a to-do list. By "anchoring" your

routine to an established habit, you make it easier to remember and incorporate.

3. Focus on Timing Over Task: Rather than setting strict deadlines for every activity, try focusing on blocks of time. For example, you might designate an hour in the morning for essential work tasks but allow yourself to work on them in any order. This flexibility within a structured timeframe allows you to adjust to the natural ebb and flow of your focus.

4. Experiment with Routine Lengths: Some people thrive on a tightly structured day, while others need only a few reliable habits to stay on track. Experiment with the length and number of routines to see what works best for you.

5. Allow for "Reset" Moments: Life is unpredictable, and routines will sometimes get interrupted. Having a "reset" activity, such as taking a few deep breaths or a quick five-minute task, can help you refocus and return to your routine.

Case Study: Olivia's Flexible Routine

Olivia, a 36-year-old graphic designer, struggled with sticking to a routine because she felt boxed in by too much structure. She eventually created a "flexible routine," where she set broad timeframes for activities instead of specific times. Her morning included an hour for personal care and breakfast, but she allowed herself to choose between exercising, reading, or journaling based on how she felt that day. For her workday, she used a 2-hour block for design projects, with built-in breaks to prevent burnout.

By giving herself choices within her routine, Olivia found a way to stay structured without feeling trapped. This flexibility allowed her to stick with her routine long-term, improving both her productivity and overall well-being.

Morning and Evening Routine Ideas

Routines are highly personal, but here are some general ideas for morning and evening routines that can help bring structure to the day:

Morning Routine Ideas:

Mindfulness Moment: Start with a few minutes of deep breathing or mindfulness to center yourself.

Top 3 Priorities: Identify three key tasks or goals for the day to create focus and direction.

Tidy-Up Ritual: Spend 5-10 minutes tidying your workspace or home environment. A clear space can lead to a clear mind.

Movement: Engage in light stretching, yoga, or a quick walk to energize your body and mind.

Evening Routine Ideas:

Reflect on the Day: Take a few minutes to review your day.

Note any accomplishments, big or small, to build positive reinforcement.

Prep for Tomorrow: Set out clothes, make a to-do list, or plan breakfast to reduce stress in the morning.

Relaxation Time: Engage in a calming activity, like reading, listening to music, or practicing gratitude.

Screen-Free Time: Limit screen use at least 30 minutes before bed to help your mind wind down.

Dealing with Routine Fatigue

One of the challenges with routines is that they can feel monotonous over time, leading to "routine fatigue." For those with ADHD, the excitement of starting a new routine might fade quickly. Here are some ways to combat this:

1. Rotate Activities: Try rotating the elements of your routine every few weeks to keep things fresh. For example, if you exercise as part of your morning routine, switch between yoga, jogging, and dance workouts to maintain interest.

2. Incorporate Rewards: Attach a small reward to each completed routine. For instance, treat yourself to your favorite coffee after your morning routine or indulge in a relaxing bath as part of your evening wind-down.

3. Change the Setting: Sometimes, a change of scenery can make all the difference. If you usually plan your day at your desk, try doing it outside or at a coffee shop for a refreshing change.

4. Give Yourself a "No Routine" Day: Once in a while, allow yourself a day off from the routine. Taking a break can make it feel new and exciting when you return to it.

Reflection

Routines offer a powerful way to bring order to the often-chaotic experience of ADHD. Emma and Olivia's stories illustrate that there's no one-size-fits-all approach; the best routines are those that fit your lifestyle and personality. Through experimentation and flexibility, you can create routines that not only support your productivity but also bring peace and stability to your day.

Remember, the key to effective routines is consistency, not perfection. Even if you miss a day or your routine doesn't go as planned, you can always return to it with a fresh start. With patience and practice, routines will become a reliable foundation that helps you navigate daily challenges with greater ease and confidence.

In the next chapter, we'll explore "Time Management Techniques That Work." From time blocking to task prioritization, we'll discuss practical ways to make the most of your time, even when ADHD tries to pull you in a dozen different directions.

Through practical tips and real-life examples, you'll learn to reclaim your time and use it effectively.

4

Time Management Techniques that Work

Time management is one of the most challenging aspects for women with ADHD. With difficulties in prioritizing, staying focused, and following through, it's easy to feel like time is slipping away. However, with the right tools and techniques, it's possible to take control of your time and make meaningful progress on your goals. This chapter will cover practical time management methods, like time blocking, the Pomodoro Technique, and prioritizing tasks in ways that align with the ADHD brain.

The Importance of Structure in Time Management

For those with ADHD, time often feels abstract — it can be difficult to gauge how long something will take or to maintain a sense of urgency. Creating structure helps bring time into focus, making it easier to manage. While too much structure can feel restrictive, finding a balance that works for you can offer the freedom to get things done without feeling overwhelmed.

Take Laura's Story: Laura, a 28-year-old social worker, struggled with time management, often arriving late to appointments and missing deadlines. She felt guilty and stressed, as her clients and colleagues depended on her. Laura knew she needed a change but didn't know where to begin. A friend suggested time blocking, and Laura gave it a try. She started by blocking specific time slots for her daily tasks, allowing her to prioritize her workload and set realistic expectations. Over time, her sense of control over her schedule improved, and her stress levels dropped.

Laura's story illustrates how even a simple technique like time blocking can make a significant impact on time management, especially when approached with ADHD-friendly strategies.

Practical Time Management Techniques

There are several time management methods that can be especially helpful for women with ADHD. Here, we'll explore a few of the most effective ones and offer tips for implementing them.

1. Time Blocking

Time blocking involves dividing your day into chunks, dedicating each block to a specific activity or type of task. For instance, you might set aside an hour in the morning for emails, followed by a two-hour block for focused work.

How to Start: Begin by identifying the major categories of tasks you need to accomplish (e.g., work, errands, self-care). Allocate specific blocks of time to each category based on your daily

TIME MANAGEMENT TECHNIQUES THAT WORK

energy levels. For example, if you're more alert in the morning, use that time for focus-intensive work.

Benefits for ADHD: Time blocking creates a predictable rhythm, making it easier to stay focused and avoid getting sidetracked. It also reduces decision fatigue, as you don't have to constantly decide what to work on next.

2. The Pomodoro Technique

The Pomodoro Technique involves working in short bursts (usually 25 minutes) followed by a 5-minute break. After four "Pomodoros," you take a longer break of 15-30 minutes.

How to Start: Set a timer for 25 minutes and focus on a single task until the timer goes off. Take a 5-minute break to recharge. Repeat the cycle three more times before taking a longer break.

Benefits for ADHD: Short, timed intervals make tasks feel less overwhelming, while regular breaks prevent burnout. The structure of this technique helps keep momentum and avoid distractions.

3. Prioritizing with the Eisenhower Matrix

The Eisenhower Matrix helps you prioritize tasks by dividing them into four categories: urgent and important, important but not urgent, urgent but not important, and neither urgent nor important.

How to Start: Write down your to-do list, then categorize each task. Focus on the urgent and important tasks first, then move on to the important but not urgent ones. Try to minimize tasks in the other two categories, as they tend to be less impactful.

Benefits for ADHD: This system helps clarify what deserves your immediate attention, making it easier to avoid getting bogged down by low-priority tasks.

4. Using Alarms and Reminders

Setting alarms and reminders can be a lifesaver, especially for recurring tasks or appointments. Many women with ADHD find it helpful to set multiple reminders leading up to a task.

How to Start: Use your phone or another device to set reminders for critical tasks. For instance, set an alarm for 10 minutes before an important meeting to give yourself time to prepare.

Benefits for ADHD: Alarms create external cues, which can help keep you on track and prevent tasks from slipping through the cracks.

5. Batching Similar Tasks

Task batching involves grouping similar activities together to complete them in one go. For example, you might set aside time to answer all your emails at once instead of sporadically throughout the day.

How to Start: Identify tasks that can be batched, such as responding to messages, preparing meals, or organizing paperwork. Dedicate a specific time block to each group of tasks.

Benefits for ADHD: Batching minimizes task-switching, which can be mentally exhausting. It also helps you build momentum as you work through similar activities.

Case Study: Jane's Structured Workday

Jane, a freelance writer and single mother, found it difficult to juggle her work and family responsibilities. She would often start writing only to get interrupted by household tasks, leading to frustration and unfinished work. After researching time management techniques, she decided to implement time blocking and the Pomodoro Technique.

Jane began by blocking out specific hours for her work and personal tasks, setting clear boundaries between them. She used the Pomodoro Technique during her work blocks, setting a timer for 25 minutes of focused writing followed by a short break. This structure gave her the focus she needed to meet deadlines without feeling overwhelmed.

As she got used to her new schedule, Jane noticed that her productivity improved, and she had more time for her family. By creating boundaries and using structured time, Jane managed to regain control over her day, finding balance between her work and home life.

Tips for Overcoming Common Time Management Struggles

Many women with ADHD face unique time management challenges, from "time blindness" to procrastination. Here are some tips to help address these specific struggles:

1. Dealing with Time Blindness: Time blindness, or the inability to gauge the passage of time accurately, is common in ADHD. Using a timer, like in the Pomodoro Technique, can provide a tangible way to track time. Visual timers, such as hourglasses or time-tracking apps, can also help you stay aware of how much time has passed.

2. Fighting Procrastination: Breaking tasks into smaller steps can reduce the mental barrier to starting. Set a timer for just 5 minutes and tell yourself you'll work on the task for that time only. Often, getting started is the hardest part, and this technique can help you push past initial resistance.

3. Avoiding "Hyper-Focus" Overload: While hyper-focus can be productive, it can also lead to burnout if you lose track of time. Setting alarms or asking a friend to check in can help you stay mindful and take breaks, avoiding the crash that sometimes follows long periods of hyper-focus.

4. Keeping a "Brain Dump" List: If new ideas or tasks keep popping into your mind, keep a notebook or app where you can jot them down. This "brain dump" allows you to capture thoughts without interrupting your focus, so you can return to them later.

Reflection

Time management can be one of the most daunting aspects of life with ADHD, but with practical tools like time blocking, the Pomodoro Technique, and prioritizing tasks, it's possible to reclaim control over your time. Laura and Jane's stories highlight the impact of structured time on productivity and mental clarity, illustrating that a few strategic adjustments can make a world of difference.

As you work to integrate these techniques, remember that progress is more important than perfection. There will be days when things don't go as planned, and that's okay. Time management is a skill that grows over time, and each small victory brings you closer to mastering it.

In the next chapter, we'll tackle the concept of decluttering and how a clear physical space can lead to a clearer mental space. Through practical tips and real-life examples, you'll learn strategies to organize your home and workspace in ways that make managing ADHD easier and more enjoyable.

5

Decluttering for Focus

For many women with ADHD, clutter is more than just a messy room or a stack of unfiled papers — it can become a source of stress and distraction that makes it difficult to focus or relax. A cluttered environment often mirrors a cluttered mind, amplifying the sense of being overwhelmed. By creating a cleaner, more organized space, you can help reduce stress and create an environment that supports your productivity. This chapter will explore practical, ADHD-friendly strategies for decluttering your home and workspace in small, manageable steps.

The Link Between Physical Space and Mental Clarity

Research shows that our physical surroundings can impact our mental health and productivity. For women with ADHD, clutter can lead to sensory overload and make it difficult to concentrate on tasks. A clear space can bring a sense of calm and clarity, making it easier to stay on track and reducing the mental fatigue associated with constant visual distractions.

Take Rachel's Story: Rachel, a 39-year-old accountant, found it impossible to focus on her work when her home was in disarray. She'd often feel anxious just walking into her living room, where piles of unopened mail and scattered paperwork greeted her. Realizing that the clutter was contributing to her stress, she decided to tackle it, one small area at a time. Over a few weeks, Rachel managed to clear out her living room and set up a simple organizational system. The difference in her mental clarity and productivity was profound.

Rachel's experience demonstrates that decluttering can be transformative for both physical and mental space, helping to reduce anxiety and create a supportive environment.

Steps to Declutter in ADHD-Friendly Increments

Decluttering can feel overwhelming, especially if there's a lot to tackle. For women with ADHD, the key is to break the process down into manageable steps, allowing for steady progress without burnout.

1. Start Small: Rather than trying to declutter an entire room, focus on a specific area, such as a single drawer or shelf. Completing a small section allows you to experience a quick win, which builds motivation to keep going.

2. Use the "One Touch" Rule: The one-touch rule means handling each item only once, making a quick decision about whether to keep, donate, or toss it. This rule minimizes rethinking and revisiting items, reducing decision fatigue.

3. Set a Timer: Decluttering doesn't have to be an hours-long task. Set a timer for 10-15 minutes and work on a specific area during that time. This technique allows you to make progress in small bursts, making the task feel more achievable.

4. Create "Zones" for Items: Assign specific places for items based on how often you use them. For instance, frequently used items should be easily accessible, while things you rarely use can be stored out of sight. Zones help maintain a sense of order and make it easier to find things when you need them.

5. Purge Regularly: Clutter has a way of creeping back in, so it's important to build decluttering into your routine. A monthly "purge session" can help keep your space organized and prevent small messes from becoming overwhelming.

Case Study: Lisa's One-Area-at-a-Time Approach

Lisa, a busy mom with two young children, felt like she was constantly surrounded by clutter. She wanted a clean, peaceful home but found it hard to stay organized. After researching ADHD-friendly organization methods, she decided to focus on one area of her house each week.

Lisa began by organizing her kitchen counter, a spot that frequently attracted clutter. She set a timer for 15 minutes each day to work on this area, purging old items and setting up a designated spot for things like keys and mail. Once the kitchen counter was under control, she moved on to her bathroom drawers, then to her entryway. Over time, Lisa's one-area-at-a-time approach transformed her home, creating a more relaxing environment without overwhelming her.

Strategies for Creating and Maintaining Order

Maintaining a clutter-free space requires routines that prevent new clutter from building up. Here are some strategies to help you create a sustainable organization system that works for the long term:

1. The "One In, One Out" Rule: For every new item you bring into your home, remove an old item. This rule can help prevent clutter from accumulating and encourages mindful purchasing.

2. Daily 5-Minute Tidy: A quick daily tidy-up can keep clutter from piling up. Spend five minutes each evening putting items back in their designated spots. This habit is especially helpful for high-traffic areas like the kitchen, bathroom, and entryway.

3. Storage Solutions That Work for You: Invest in storage solutions that match your needs and preferences. Clear bins, baskets, and drawer dividers can make it easier to stay organized. Labeling can also help, making it easy to find items and return them to their rightful place.

4. Donate Regularly: Set up a donation box in your home, adding items you no longer need as you come across them. When the box is full, take it to a donation center. This process keeps things moving out of your space and makes letting go of items less overwhelming.

5. Create "Drop Zones" for Daily Essentials: Drop zones are

designated spots for frequently used items, like keys, wallets, and phones. This helps prevent them from getting lost and reduces the clutter that can accumulate from leaving items in random places.

Dealing with Sentimental Clutter

For many women with ADHD, parting with sentimental items can be challenging. These items often hold memories and emotional attachments, making it hard to let them go. Here are some ways to manage sentimental clutter without feeling like you're losing part of your past:

1. Keep the Best, Let Go of the Rest: Focus on keeping a select few items that hold the most meaning. Instead of holding onto a box of old cards, for instance, choose just a few that mean the most to you.

2. Take Photos: For items that are too bulky to keep, consider taking photos. You can still keep the memory without needing to hold onto the physical item.

3. Create a Memory Box: Set aside a small box specifically for sentimental items. When it's full, revisit the items and decide if you still need to keep everything inside. This method helps contain sentimental items to a manageable space.

Reflection

Decluttering may seem like a daunting task, but for women with ADHD, a clear space can bring a clear mind. Rachel and Lisa's stories highlight the power of small, consistent efforts in transforming a cluttered environment into one that supports mental and emotional well-being. By breaking the process down into manageable steps and creating sustainable habits, you can make decluttering a regular part of your life.

As you tackle each area of your space, remember that progress is more important than perfection. Even small changes can lead to big improvements in focus, productivity, and peace of mind. By creating a space that reflects clarity and organization, you can reduce distractions and feel more in control.

In the next chapter, we'll explore "Organizing with Digital Tools," focusing on apps and technology that can help manage tasks, reminders, and priorities. You'll learn about ADHD-friendly tools that make organization easier, helping you stay on top of your responsibilities without feeling overwhelmed.

6

Organising with Digital Tools

In today's world, technology offers powerful tools that can make managing life with ADHD easier and more efficient. From apps that help track tasks and set reminders to digital calendars and note-taking platforms, digital tools can be a game-changer for staying organized and reducing mental load. This chapter will explore practical ways to use digital tools for organization and share tips on finding the right apps and methods for your unique needs.

The Benefits of Digital Organization

For women with ADHD, digital tools can provide external structure and accountability, helping bridge gaps in memory, time management, and focus. Digital tools allow you to keep track of everything in one place, freeing up mental space and reducing stress. A well-organized digital system also makes it easier to prioritize tasks, plan your day, and minimize the anxiety that comes from forgetting important commitments.

Consider Sophia's Story: Sophia, a 30-year-old freelance writer, constantly struggled with keeping track of deadlines and appointments. She'd often forget meetings or double-book herself, leading to lost clients and unnecessary stress. A friend introduced her to digital organization tools, and Sophia decided to give them a try. She began using a task management app and a digital calendar to organize her work and personal life. By setting reminders and creating a clear daily plan, Sophia transformed her workflow and regained control over her time.

Sophia's experience shows that digital tools, when used thoughtfully, can create a streamlined structure that supports productivity and minimizes stress.

Digital Tools to Help You Stay Organized

There are countless digital tools available, each with unique features that cater to different organizational needs. Here are some of the most effective types of tools for ADHD-friendly organization:

1. Task Management Apps

Task management apps like Todoist, Trello, or Microsoft To-Do help you break down tasks into manageable steps, set priorities, and track progress. Many apps allow you to create different projects or lists, making it easier to organize tasks by category.

How to Use: Begin by listing all your tasks in one place, then categorize them into projects (e.g., work, personal, errands). Set due dates for tasks and use reminders for high-priority items.

Benefits for ADHD: Task management apps allow you to offload your mental to-do list, making it easier to remember everything and focus on one task at a time.

2. Digital Calendars

Digital calendars like Google Calendar or Outlook provide a central location for managing appointments, deadlines, and recurring events. Many digital calendars also offer notification options and allow you to share events with others.

How to Use: Schedule both work and personal commitments on the same calendar to avoid double-booking. Set alerts 10-15 minutes before important appointments to ensure you have enough time to prepare.

Benefits for ADHD: A digital calendar provides a visual overview of your schedule, helping you manage your time more effectively and avoid missing important events.

3. Reminder Apps

For quick reminders and one-off tasks, apps like Apple Reminders or Google Keep can be helpful. They allow you to set short-term reminders without cluttering your main to-do list or calendar.

How to Use: Use reminder apps for small tasks like "call the doctor" or "pay the electric bill." Set notifications at the ideal time of day to ensure you'll be able to take action.

Benefits for ADHD: Quick reminders help you stay on top of small tasks that are easy to forget, minimizing last-minute rushes and forgotten responsibilities.

4. Note-Taking Apps

Note-taking apps like Evernote, OneNote, or Notion are invaluable for organizing ideas, keeping track of information, and managing long-term projects. They allow you to store information in a digital format that's easy to access and search.

How to Use: Use note-taking apps to record meeting notes, brainstorming ideas, or any information you might need later. Create separate notebooks or folders for different topics.

Benefits for ADHD: A central place for notes reduces mental clutter and allows you to retrieve information quickly, helping you stay organized and focused on your tasks.

5. Time-Tracking Tools

Time-tracking tools like Toggl or RescueTime can help you monitor how you're spending your time. This is especially useful for identifying where you may be losing focus or spending too much time on low-priority tasks.

How to Use: Start by tracking your time for one week to get a baseline understanding of your work habits. Review the data to identify patterns and adjust your schedule accordingly.

Benefits for ADHD: Time-tracking tools provide concrete data on how you spend your time, making it easier to set goals and improve productivity without relying on guesswork.

Case Study: Mia's Digital Toolbox

Mia, a 45-year-old project manager, juggled multiple responsibilities at work and home. She felt constantly overwhelmed, often forgetting important deadlines and struggling to manage her workload. Mia decided to experiment with digital tools to create a more organized system.

She began with a digital calendar, where she entered all her meetings, deadlines, and family commitments. She then started using Trello to organize her work tasks by project, setting due dates for each step. For her personal tasks, Mia used Apple Reminders to manage her daily errands and routine responsibilities.

Over time, Mia found her "digital toolbox" gave her a clearer sense of control and direction. Her calendar provided a visual overview of her schedule, while Trello kept her work tasks organized and manageable. The reminder app helped her stay on top of personal responsibilities without overwhelming her main task list. Mia's digital system gave her the structure she needed to stay on track, reduce stress, and balance her work and personal life effectively.

Tips for Finding the Right Digital Tools

The right digital tools can make a world of difference in organizing life with ADHD, but finding the best options for your unique needs requires experimentation. Here are some tips to help you get started:

1. Start Simple: Don't overwhelm yourself with too many tools at once. Begin with one or two core tools, such as a task manager and calendar, and gradually add others as needed.

2. Look for ADHD-Friendly Features: Features like reminders, color-coding, and visual task boards can make tools more ADHD-friendly. Prioritize apps with these features to make your digital system more intuitive.

3. Customize to Fit Your Lifestyle: Many digital tools are highly customizable. Experiment with different layouts, notification settings, and organization methods to find what works best for you.

4. Set Aside Time for "Digital Maintenance": Just like a physical space, digital spaces need regular upkeep. Set aside time each week to review and update your to-do list, calendar, and notes to ensure they stay organized.

5. Remember It's OK to Switch Tools: Don't feel obligated to stick with a tool that isn't working for you. It's okay to experiment until you find the best fit. Many women with ADHD find that their organizational needs change over time, so revisiting your toolset periodically can be helpful.

Reflection

Digital tools offer endless possibilities for creating a structured, ADHD-friendly organizational system. Sophia and Mia's stories show how a few carefully chosen tools can reduce stress, improve time management, and bring greater clarity to daily life. By choosing the right tools and tailoring them to your needs, you can create a streamlined system that supports your goals and allows you to thrive.

As you explore the world of digital organization, remember that it's about progress, not perfection. Start with simple steps, experiment, and gradually build a digital organization system that works for you.

In the next chapter, we'll delve into "Managing Finances with ADHD." Many women with ADHD find financial management challenging, but with practical budgeting and expense-tracking strategies, it's possible to take control of your finances and reduce financial stress. Through practical tips and real-life examples, you'll learn how to simplify financial management and make it ADHD-friendly.

7

Managing Finances with ADHD

Financial management can be a significant challenge for women with ADHD. Keeping track of bills, budgeting, and managing expenses often requires a level of organization and consistency that can feel overwhelming. Financial stress can amplify ADHD symptoms, creating a cycle of anxiety and avoidance. However, with the right tools and strategies, it's possible to take control of your finances, build confidence, and reduce stress. This chapter will provide practical, ADHD-friendly methods for budgeting, tracking expenses, and managing bills effectively.

The Unique Financial Challenges for Women with ADHD

For many women with ADHD, managing money comes with unique challenges. Impulsivity can lead to overspending, while difficulties with organization and time management can result in late payments and missed bills. Moreover, the tendency to feel overwhelmed by complex tasks can make budgeting and expense tracking seem daunting. Addressing these challenges with simple, ADHD-friendly systems can make financial management more approachable and sustainable.

Consider Ella's Story: Ella, a 33-year-old nurse, struggled to keep her finances organized. She often avoided looking at her bank account, leading to unplanned overdrafts and credit card debt. The stress of her finances affected her mental health and made her feel constantly anxious. Determined to make a change, Ella sought out tools and strategies that suited her ADHD needs. She began using a budgeting app with automatic alerts and set up regular "money check-ins" to review her spending. With time, Ella gained control over her finances, reduced her debt, and felt empowered by her progress.

Ella's experience shows that by using the right tools and establishing small routines, it's possible to take control of your finances even if it feels overwhelming at first.

Step-by-Step Strategies for Managing Finances

1. Create a Simple Budgeting System

A budget is a roadmap for your finances, helping you plan where your money goes each month. For women with ADHD, a straightforward budget with a few key categories can make financial planning more manageable.

How to Start: Identify a few essential categories, such as rent/mortgage, groceries, transportation, and entertainment. Use a budgeting app like You Need a Budget (YNAB), Mint, or Goodbudget to track your spending and set limits for each category.

Benefits for ADHD: Apps with visual breakdowns and automatic tracking simplify the budgeting process and provide a clear picture of where your money is going.

2. Use Automatic Bill Pay and Reminders

Setting up automatic payments for recurring bills, like rent, utilities, and credit card payments, can reduce the risk of late fees and missed payments. Most banking apps and financial management tools also offer reminders for non-automated bills.

How to Start: Set up automatic payments for as many bills as possible through your bank or service providers. For bills that can't be automated, use reminders on your phone or a financial app to prompt you when they're due.

Benefits for ADHD: Automating bills reduces the number of tasks you need to remember each month, allowing you to focus on other financial priorities.

3. Track Your Spending Weekly

Tracking spending helps prevent surprises at the end of the month and ensures you stay within your budget. For those with ADHD, a weekly "money check-in" can make it easier to manage expenses without feeling overwhelmed by a month's worth of data.

How to Start: Choose a specific day each week to review your spending. Use a budgeting app or a simple spreadsheet to categorize your expenses and check if you're staying within your budget.

Benefits for ADHD: Weekly tracking makes financial manage-ment feel less daunting, helping you catch potential issues early and make adjustments as needed.

4. Set Small, Achievable Savings Goals

Building savings can feel overwhelming, but breaking it down into smaller goals can make it more manageable. Start with a modest goal, such as saving a specific amount each month for an emergency fund, a vacation, or a purchase you're planning.

How to Start: Decide on a savings amount that feels achievable, even if it's small. Open a separate savings account, and consider setting up automatic transfers to make saving consistent.

Benefits for ADHD: Small goals create momentum and allow you to see tangible progress, which can motivate you to keep saving over time.

5. Use Cash Envelopes for Discretionary Spending

For discretionary spending categories like dining out, enter-tainment, or shopping, the cash envelope system can provide a visual way to stay within budget. Once the cash is gone, you know you've reached your limit for the month.

How to Start: Decide on an amount for each discretionary category, withdraw the cash, and place it in envelopes labeled for each purpose. Use cash for these expenses until the envelope is empty.

Benefits for ADHD: Physical cash provides a clear, tactile limit, helping prevent overspending and making budgeting feel more concrete.

Case Study: Sarah's Financial Routine

Sarah, a 41-year-old graphic designer, felt like she was always scrambling to manage her finances. She frequently forgot bill payments, resulting in fees that ate into her budget. Frustrated, she researched ADHD-friendly financial strategies and decided to try a weekly "money check-in" routine and cash envelopes for her discretionary spending.

Every Sunday, Sarah reviewed her bank account, checked her budgeting app, and updated her cash envelopes. This routine provided structure and made her feel more in control. By the end of the month, Sarah noticed that her spending was more aligned with her goals, and she hadn't incurred any late fees. Over time, her financial routine became a habit, giving her peace of mind and reducing her financial anxiety.

Tips for Building Sustainable Financial Habits

Building lasting financial habits is key to managing finances effectively. Here are some strategies to help sustain your progress:

1. Reward Yourself for Staying on Track: Set small rewards for sticking to your budget or reaching savings goals. A small treat, like a favorite snack or a relaxing activity, can help reinforce positive financial habits.

2. Simplify with Fewer Accounts: Having multiple accounts or credit cards can complicate financial management. Try to consolidate accounts where possible to make tracking expenses easier.

3. Make Financial Check-Ins Routine: Set a regular time each week or month to review your finances. This check-in routine helps you stay aware of your spending and make adjustments before problems arise.

4. Build a Buffer for Unexpected Expenses: Life is unpredictable, and unexpected expenses can throw off your budget. Aim to keep a small buffer in your checking account or savings to cover surprises, like a car repair or medical bill.

5. Seek Support if Needed: If you find financial management particularly challenging, consider seeking support from a financial coach or planner. Many professionals specialize in ADHD-friendly financial strategies and can provide tailored guidance.

Reflection

Managing finances can be one of the most challenging aspects of life with ADHD, but it's also one of the most empowering. Ella and Sarah's stories illustrate that with small, consistent steps, it's possible to build financial habits that support stability and reduce stress. By creating routines, using technology, and setting achievable goals, you can regain control of your finances and build confidence in your financial future.

As you implement these strategies, remember that it's okay to make mistakes. Financial management is a learning process, and each step brings you closer to financial security and peace of mind.

In the next chapter, we'll explore "Relationships and ADHD." Managing ADHD-related challenges in relationships, whether with partners, family, or friends, requires understanding, communication, and self-awareness. Through real-life stories and practical tips, you'll learn strategies to navigate relationship dynamics and build stronger, more supportive connections.

8

Relationships and ADHD

Relationships can be deeply rewarding yet challenging, especially for women with ADHD. ADHD symptoms — like impulsivity, forgetfulness, and emotional sensitivity — can impact communication, trust, and understanding between partners, family members, and friends. However, with open communication, empathy, and strategies tailored to ADHD challenges, it's possible to build strong, supportive relationships. This chapter will explore practical ways to manage ADHD in relationships and foster deeper connections with loved ones.

Understanding ADHD's Impact on Relationships

Women with ADHD often face unique struggles in relationships. Emotional intensity, impulsivity, and forgetfulness can sometimes be misinterpreted, leading to frustration and misunderstandings. For many, guilt and shame around ADHD symptoms may further complicate relationships, making it difficult to ask for support or communicate openly.

Consider Lily's Story: Lily, a 36-year-old marketing execu-tive, often found herself arguing with her partner, Sam, over seemingly small things. She would forget plans, lose track of time, or get so engrossed in a project that she wouldn't respond to messages for hours. Sam felt neglected, while Lily felt misunderstood and embarrassed by her forgetfulness. After researching ADHD's impact on relationships, Lily and Sam decided to work on better communication and understanding. Lily began using reminders for plans, and Sam learned to interpret some behaviors as ADHD-related, not as signs of disinterest.

Lily's experience shows that awareness and communication can go a long way in strengthening relationships and helping both partners feel supported and understood.

Practical Tips for Managing ADHD in Relationships

1. Communicate Openly About ADHD

Many partners and family members may not fully understand ADHD or may have misconceptions about it. Openly discussing ADHD, its symptoms, and how it impacts daily life can help clear up misunderstandings and build empathy.

How to Start: Begin with a calm, honest conversation about how ADHD affects your behavior. Use specific examples to illustrate challenges, such as "I often lose track of time, which is why I may seem late or distracted."

Benefits for ADHD: Open communication fosters empathy,

helping your loved ones understand that certain behaviors stem from ADHD, not a lack of interest or care.

2. Set Clear Expectations and Boundaries

ADHD can make it hard to manage time, plan, or stick to commitments. Setting clear expectations for routines, schedules, or responsibilities helps prevent misunderstandings and builds trust.

How to Start: Work with your partner or family members to create a shared schedule or list of responsibilities. Be transparent about areas where you may need support or reminders.

Benefits for ADHD: Clear expectations reduce miscommunication, allowing both parties to understand and respect each other's needs.

3. Use Reminders and Shared Calendars

Using tools like shared calendars, reminders, or scheduling apps can help you stay on top of plans and commitments. Shared calendars allow both you and your partner to see upcoming events and deadlines, which reduces the mental load of remembering everything.

How to Start: Use a calendar app like Google Calendar or an organization tool like Trello. Create shared events and set reminders to help you stay on track.

Benefits for ADHD: External reminders take pressure off memory, helping you stay organized and respectful of your loved one's time and expectations.

4. Practice Active Listening and Empathy

ADHD can sometimes make it challenging to stay present in conversations, especially during emotional discussions. Practicing active listening — making a conscious effort to hear and understand your partner's feelings — helps strengthen your connection.

How to Start: When your partner is speaking, focus on listening without interrupting. Acknowledge their feelings by summarizing what they've said and responding with empathy.

Benefits for ADHD: Active listening builds trust and respect, showing your partner that you value their thoughts and emotions, even if you're sometimes prone to distraction.

5. Work Together to Find Solutions

Relationships work best when both parties support each other's growth. When challenges arise, approach them as a team, focusing on solutions rather than blame.

How to Start: Frame conversations around solutions rather than focusing on what went wrong. For example, if you forgot an important date, acknowledge it, apologize, and discuss ways to prevent it from happening in the future.

Benefits for ADHD: Working together to find solutions strengthens bonds and reduces feelings of shame or inadequacy, creating a healthier, more supportive dynamic.

Case Study: Emma and Mike's Communication Strategies

Emma, a 40-year-old teacher, often felt frustrated with her husband, Mike, who didn't understand her ADHD symptoms. She would get easily overwhelmed by household chores, leaving things half-done or forgetting entirely. Mike felt like he was taking on the bulk of household responsibilities and became resentful.

After some difficult conversations, Emma and Mike agreed to try new communication strategies. Emma created a task list to track her household responsibilities, and Mike checked in with her at the end of each week to discuss any areas where she might need help. Over time, this collaborative approach eased their tension, with Mike feeling more involved and Emma feeling less judged. Their relationship improved as they both developed empathy for each other's challenges.

Self-Care and Boundaries in Relationships

Managing ADHD in relationships also involves taking care of yourself. It's essential to practice self-compassion and set boundaries to protect your mental health and well-being.

1. Practice Self-Compassion: Many women with ADHD feel guilt or shame over their symptoms, which can lead to self-criticism. Treat yourself with kindness and recognize that ADHD is part of who you are, not a flaw or shortcoming.

2. Set Boundaries: It's okay to set boundaries to protect your energy and focus. If you need quiet time to concentrate or un-wind, communicate this to your loved ones so they understand your needs.

3. Celebrate Small Wins Together: Recognize and celebrate progress, no matter how small. For example, if you successfully follow through on a plan or complete a shared goal, take a moment to acknowledge and appreciate the achievement together.

Reflection

Relationships can be complex, especially when managing ADHD, but with open communication, empathy, and practical strate-gies, they can become sources of support and joy. Lily and Emma's stories illustrate how understanding, clear expecta-tions, and teamwork can strengthen bonds, making relation-ships more resilient and fulfilling.

Remember, ADHD is just one part of who you are. By embrac-ing honest communication, setting boundaries, and working together to overcome challenges, you and your loved ones can build connections that bring stability, understanding, and mutual respect.

In the next chapter, we'll discuss "Self-Care and Mental Health," focusing on self-care practices that help manage stress, boost mental resilience, and improve focus. Through practical self-care strategies and real-life examples, you'll learn how to prioritize your well-being while managing life with ADHD.

9

Self Care and Mental Health

Self-care is an essential aspect of managing ADHD, especially for women who often juggle multiple roles and responsibilities. ADHD can intensify stress and make it challenging to balance personal needs with daily obligations, leading to burnout and mental fatigue. Prioritizing self-care and mental health practices helps manage ADHD symptoms, reduce stress, and build resilience. This chapter will explore practical self-care strategies that are ADHD-friendly and offer tips for building a routine that supports mental and emotional well-being.

Why Self-Care Is Vital for Women with ADHD

Women with ADHD often experience higher levels of stress and anxiety, especially when trying to meet expectations at work, at home, and in relationships. The mental energy required to manage ADHD can be exhausting, and without regular self-care, it's easy to feel overwhelmed or defeated. Incorporating self-care practices into daily life can boost focus, improve mood, and increase the capacity to handle challenges.

Consider Hannah's Story: Hannah, a 38-year-old mother and nurse, felt constantly drained by her responsibilities at work and home. She struggled with guilt, feeling she was never doing "enough," and rarely took time for herself. After a particularly difficult month, Hannah's friend suggested prioritizing self-care to manage stress. Hannah began by setting aside 10 minutes each morning for deep breathing and journaling, followed by a few minutes of gentle stretching. Gradually, she noticed an improvement in her mood and energy levels, and her ADHD symptoms became more manageable.

Hannah's journey demonstrates that even small, consistent self-care practices can have a powerful impact on mental health, helping to counterbalance the challenges of ADHD.

Self-Care Practices to Support Mental Health

1. Mindfulness and Meditation

Mindfulness practices, like meditation or deep breathing, can help calm a racing mind and improve focus. For women with ADHD, taking a few minutes to practice mindfulness each day can reduce anxiety, enhance self-awareness, and increase resilience.

How to Start: Begin with just 3-5 minutes of mindful breathing each morning. Apps like Headspace, Calm, or Insight Timer offer guided meditations that are short and easy to follow.

Benefits for ADHD: Mindfulness can help reduce impulsivity, improve emotional regulation, and provide a grounding effect, helping you stay focused and calm in challenging situations.

2. Exercise and Movement

Regular physical activity can significantly impact ADHD symptoms by releasing endorphins, improving focus, and reducing anxiety. Exercise doesn't have to be intense; even a short walk or gentle stretching can help boost your mood and energy.

How to Start: Find a form of movement you enjoy, whether it's dancing, yoga, or a brisk walk. Aim for 15-30 minutes a day, starting with just a few days a week.

Benefits for ADHD: Exercise provides a healthy outlet for excess energy, improves cognitive function, and reduces the mental fog that often accompanies ADHD.

3. Prioritizing Sleep

Sleep is essential for mental and physical health, but ADHD can make it difficult to establish a consistent sleep routine. Prioritizing good sleep hygiene can improve focus, mood, and energy levels, making it easier to manage ADHD symptoms.

How to Start: Set a regular bedtime, limit screen time an hour before bed, and create a calming bedtime routine. Apps like Sleep Cycle can help track your sleep patterns.

Benefits for ADHD: Quality sleep improves memory, attention, and emotional regulation, making it easier to handle daily tasks with clarity and focus.

4. Setting Realistic Goals and Celebrating Progress

Many women with ADHD set high expectations for themselves, leading to feelings of inadequacy. Setting small, realistic goals and celebrating achievements, no matter how small, can build self-confidence and reduce stress.

How to Start: Choose one or two manageable goals each day, such as completing a task or taking time to rest. When you accomplish a goal, take a moment to celebrate it — even a small acknowledgment can boost morale.

Benefits for ADHD: Celebrating progress reinforces positive habits, builds confidence, and helps create a sense of accomplishment.

5. Engaging in Hobbies and Creative Outlets

Pursuing hobbies and creative activities provides a break from daily stress and allows for self-expression. Activities like drawing, painting, gardening, or crafting can be therapeutic, helping to release tension and spark joy.

How to Start: Set aside 15-30 minutes a few times a week for a hobby or activity you enjoy. Try new creative outlets and find what resonates with you.

Benefits for ADHD: Hobbies offer a way to focus on enjoyable tasks, reduce anxiety, and provide a sense of purpose beyond daily responsibilities.

Case Study: Sophia's Self-Care Routine

Sophia, a 42-year-old lawyer, struggled with feeling burned out and overwhelmed. Balancing a demanding career with personal commitments left her exhausted, and her ADHD symptoms felt more pronounced during high-stress periods. Realizing she needed a change, Sophia created a self-care routine focused on small but meaningful practices.

She started each morning with 10 minutes of meditation and 15 minutes of stretching. In the evenings, she wrote in a gratitude journal, listing three things she was grateful for that day. She also made time each week for her favorite hobby, painting. Over time, Sophia found that these small practices made a substantial difference, helping her manage stress, boost her focus, and feel more balanced.

Building a Self-Care Routine that Works for You

1. Start Small: Introducing too many self-care practices at once can feel overwhelming. Start with one or two simple practices that you can incorporate into your daily routine, like deep breathing or a short walk.

2. Listen to Your Body and Mind: Self-care isn't one-size-fits-all. Tune into your needs and adjust your routine as necessary. Some days you may need a quiet moment alone, while other days, a social connection might be what you need most.

3. Establish Consistency, Not Perfection: Self-care routines don't have to be perfect. It's okay if you miss a day or need

to adjust your practices. Consistency is more important than perfection; aim to incorporate self-care regularly, even if it's in small doses.

4. Prioritize What Brings You Joy and Calm: Self-care should feel nourishing, not like another chore. Focus on activities that genuinely bring you joy, relaxation, or a sense of accomplishment.

5. Ask for Support When Needed: Don't hesitate to reach out for support from friends, family, or mental health professionals if you're struggling. Sometimes, self-care means seeking help from others to lighten your load.

Reflection

Self-care is a vital part of managing ADHD, supporting mental and emotional resilience. Hannah and Sophia's stories show that small, consistent practices can make a substantial difference in managing stress and improving well-being. By incorporating mindfulness, movement, sleep, and creative outlets, you can create a self-care routine that aligns with your unique needs and lifestyle.

As you explore self-care practices, remember that this journey is about finding balance and honoring yourself. Self-care allows you to show up more fully in all areas of your life, helping you manage ADHD with compassion and strength.

In the final chapter, we'll discuss "Embracing Your Unique ADHD Strengths." ADHD brings both challenges and strengths, and by recognizing and leveraging your unique abilities, you can build a life filled with purpose and accomplishment. Through real-life examples and practical tips, you'll learn how to embrace the gifts of ADHD and turn them into assets for your personal and professional life.

10

Embrace your Unique ADHD Strengths

ADHD is often associated with challenges, but it also brings unique strengths. Many women with ADHD possess exceptional creativity, resilience, adaptability, and the ability to hyper-focus when truly engaged. By embracing and leveraging these strengths, you can transform perceived "weaknesses" into assets. This final chapter focuses on identifying your unique abilities, building confidence, and finding ways to harness these strengths in both personal and professional life.

Recognizing ADHD Strengths

While ADHD symptoms can be challenging, they also create qualities that are beneficial in many aspects of life. Here are a few common strengths associated with ADHD:

1. Creativity and Out-of-the-Box Thinking: People with ADHD often excel at thinking creatively and generating innovative ideas. This can be a valuable asset in fields that require problem-solving and fresh perspectives.

2. Hyper-Focus: Though ADHD can make it difficult to focus on mundane tasks, many with ADHD experience hyper-focus — intense focus on tasks that are engaging or meaningful. This ability can lead to deep dives into topics, fostering expertise and creative breakthroughs.

3. Resilience: Living with ADHD often involves overcoming obstacles, building resilience, and adapting to unexpected challenges. Many women with ADHD are highly adaptable and resourceful, able to pivot quickly in changing situations.

4. High Energy and Enthusiasm: Many women with ADHD possess a high level of enthusiasm and energy, which can be contagious and inspiring. This quality often makes them natural leaders or motivators within teams.

5. Empathy and Sensitivity: ADHD can heighten emotional sensitivity, which, when managed well, can become an asset. Empathy and sensitivity allow for strong interpersonal skills, making those with ADHD attuned to the emotions and needs of others.

Case Study: Clara's Journey of Embracing Her Strengths

Clara, a 35-year-old designer, once saw her ADHD as a constant source of frustration. She struggled with staying organized, keeping up with deadlines, and managing her emotions. However, with the help of a coach, Clara started to reframe her ADHD-related traits as strengths rather than weaknesses.

Clara's creativity, she realized, was her biggest asset in her work. She approached each design project with a unique perspective, which quickly set her apart in her field. Her empathy and enthusiasm made her a team favorite, as colleagues often turned to her for support and fresh ideas. By focusing on her strengths rather than her challenges, Clara transformed her career and built confidence in her abilities.

Practical Ways to Leverage Your ADHD Strengths

1. Identify Your Strengths

Begin by listing qualities or traits you appreciate about yourself, even if they don't seem like "traditional" strengths. Reflect on times when these traits helped you succeed or added value to your life.

How to Start: Write down five qualities you're proud of or times when your ADHD traits turned out to be assets. This list can serve as a reminder of your abilities and a source of motivation during challenging times.

Benefits for ADHD: Acknowledging your strengths helps shift focus from perceived weaknesses to the valuable qualities you bring to the table.

2. Align Your Career with Your Strengths

Many women with ADHD find success in careers that allow for creativity, variety, and hands-on work. Identifying roles that align with your strengths can lead to greater fulfillment and success.

How to Start: Reflect on what aspects of your work energize you and what environments support your best self. Consider roles that value innovation, adaptability, or empathy — all strengths often associated with ADHD.

Benefits for ADHD: Working in a role that suits your natural strengths reduces stress and enhances motivation, creating a more ADHD-friendly work experience.

3. Use Hyper-Focus to Your Advantage

Hyper-focus can be incredibly powerful when directed toward productive or creative tasks. While it's essential to balance hyper-focus with breaks, this ability can be leveraged for deep work, learning, or creative pursuits.

How to Start: Set specific, meaningful goals to channel your hyper-focus productively. When you're in a state of hyper-focus, aim to work on tasks that align with your strengths or passions.

Benefits for ADHD: Hyper-focus allows for concentrated, un-interrupted work, helping you achieve significant progress on projects you care about.

4. Build a Support Network that Celebrates Your Strengths

Surrounding yourself with people who recognize and appreciate your strengths can help you stay motivated and confident.

Positive reinforcement from loved ones, friends, or mentors can be a powerful reminder of your abilities.

How to Start: Seek out relationships and communities that value and celebrate your strengths. This might include joining ADHD support groups, finding a mentor, or cultivating friendships with those who recognize your unique talents.

Benefits for ADHD: A supportive network builds confidence, provides encouragement, and offers perspective when you're feeling challenged.

5. Practice Self-Acceptance and Self-Compassion

Embracing ADHD means acknowledging both strengths and struggles. Practicing self-compassion and accepting yourself fully helps you build resilience and approach life with a positive, balanced mindset.

How to Start: Incorporate daily affirmations or reflective journaling to acknowledge and appreciate your unique qualities. Reframe challenges as opportunities for growth, and celebrate progress without focusing on perfection.

Benefits for ADHD: Self-acceptance empowers you to move beyond self-criticism, allowing you to approach challenges with confidence and a solution-oriented mindset.

Reflection on Embracing ADHD Strengths

Embracing ADHD means celebrating your unique traits while finding practical ways to manage the associated challenges. Clara's story illustrates the transformation that can occur when you choose to focus on your strengths, using them as tools to build confidence, foster growth, and contribute positively to your personal and professional life.

By identifying your strengths, finding ways to align your work and life with them, and practicing self-acceptance, you can unlock the full potential of your ADHD. This approach transforms ADHD from a barrier into a unique set of assets that enhance your ability to succeed.

Moving Forward

As we conclude this book, remember that ADHD is not a limitation but a part of who you are — a source of creativity, empathy, and resilience. The strategies, tools, and insights you've explored throughout these chapters are here to empower you to live a life filled with purpose, organization, and self-confidence.

Each chapter has offered practical ways to work with, rather than against, your ADHD, helping you create a supportive environment, routines, financial management strategies, and relationships that nurture your growth. While the journey with ADHD may have its ups and downs, remember that each step forward is a step toward greater self-awareness, fulfillment, and a life that celebrates your unique gifts.

By embracing your ADHD strengths and managing challenges

with compassion, you're equipped to thrive — creating a life that reflects your values, passions, and potential. Moving forward, may you continue to build on these strengths, support yourself with kindness, and live fully as the remarkable person you are.